Chérif SHUKURU KABERUKA

PEDIATRIC NURSING

Chérif SHUKURU KABERUKA

PEDIATRIC NURSING

Quick actions by the pediatric nurse

ScienciaScripts

Imprint

Cover image: www.ingimage.com

This book is a translation from the original published under ISBN 978-620-3-45889-3.

Publisher:
Sciencia Scripts
is a trademark of
Dodo Books Indian Ocean Ltd. and OmniScriptum S.R.L publishing group

120 High Road, East Finchley, London, N2 9ED, United Kingdom
Str. Armeneasca 28/1, office 1, Chisinau MD-2012, Republic of Moldova, Europe
Printed at: see last page
ISBN: 978-620-6-51045-1

PAEDIATRIC NURSING

Foreword

Nursing in paediatrics" is intended for students of general care and those of paediatrics, adapted to the curriculum of higher and university education in the Democratic Republic of Congo.

The originality of this book lies in the pathologies selected, but also in the examples we have cited which reflect the reality on the ground, the pathologies often encountered in our health facilities, in the Democratic Republic of Congo .

By reading this book, learners will be able to understand and interpret the common pathologies that are frequently encountered in our hospitals, and will be shown the role of the nurse and the actions required in paediatrics in general, and in the Democratic Republic of Congo in particular.

Nursing in Paediatrics consists of twelve chapters and a general introduction:

- The introduction focuses on the aims of paediatric nursing, definitions of key concepts, childhood illnesses, the organisation of the CPS service, paediatrics and the characteristics of paediatric care, the roles of the paediatric nurse and paediatric doses.
- The first chapter deals with nursing care in **neonatology**
- The second chapter deals with nursing care for respiratory diseases in children.
- The third chapter is based on nursing care for disorders of the digestive tract in children.
- The fourth chapter is based on nursing care for cardiovascular conditions in children
- Chapter five deals with diseases of the nervous system in children
- The sixth chapter deals with blood diseases
- Chapter seven deals with trauma in children
- The eighth chapter deals with general infectious diseases in children
- The ninth chapter deals with endocrine diseases
- The tenth chapter deals with the management of acute malnutrition in children.
- Chapter eleven deals with urogenital infections in children.
- The twelfth chapter deals with PMTCT and children with HIV.

We would like to express our gratitude to our supervisors: Prof DUNIA MASTAKI Jean, CT Affable IZANDENGERA, Dr BIZIMUNGU MUTAZIHARA Jean-Claude, CT TITI MAHESHE, CT Fabien KIZUNGU, CT Patrick MALISAWA, Ass Modeste NFITUMUKIZA NTIBESHE and Prof Elias SEMAJERI, not forgetting our students, whose guidance helped us to improve this module.

Table of contents

GENERAL INTRODUCTION

0.1.OBJECTIVES OF THE ECU

0.1.1.GENERAL OBJECTIVE

The student will be able to apply basic nursing correctly to all sick children and according to the new IMCI strategy.

0.1.2.SPECIFIC OBJECTIVES

At the end of this course, the regular and punctual student who has followed it attentively will be able to :

1. Carrying out a clinical examination in children;
2. Providing effective nursing care ;
3. Observing and analysing the child in order to identify disturbed basic needs and respond to them effectively;

0.2. COURSE OUTLINE

- General introduction
- Chapter One: Neonatal Nursing Care
- Chapter two: Nursing care for respiratory diseases in children.
- Chapter three: nursing care for disorders of the digestive tract in children.
- Chapter four: Nursing care for cardiovascular diseases
- Chapter five: Diseases of the nervous system
- Chapter six: Blood diseases
- Chapter Seven: Childhood trauma
- Chapter eight: General infectious diseases in children
- Chapter Nine: Endocrine Diseases
- Chapter ten: Management of acute malnutrition
- Chapter eleven: Urogenital infections in children
- Chapter Twelve: PMTCT and children with HIV

0.3 DEFINITION OF KEY CONCEPTS

0.3.1. NURSING

Nursing is the set of actions carried out by a nurse to respond to the disturbed needs of the patient.

The nurse is the first person to receive the patient in hospital, and must greet them with love and listen attentively, while avoiding distractions.

When a patient comes to us, their health has deteriorated and all their needs have been disrupted.

This is why nurses must seek to satisfy these needs, replacing the patient's position by carrying out their work as if they were doing it themselves. For example,

VIRGINIA HENDERSON believes that the role of the nurse is to help the sick person recover their health or die with dignity.
It classified human needs in order of importance as follows:

1. Breathe normally ;
2. Eat and drink as required;
3. Eliminate by all means of elimination;
4. Moving around and maintaining good posture;
5. Rest and sleep
6. Dress appropriately ;
7. Maintain body temperature within normal limits;
8. Be clean, look good and protect your skin;
9. Avoiding accident risks for patients and accident risks for others
10. Being able to communicate
11. Practising your religion according to your beliefs
12. Keeping busy so you feel useful
13. Create creative activities in a variety of forms.
14. Learning, discovering and satisfying a healthy curiosity.

O.3.2. IMCI

a. Definition

IMCI is a programme developed by the WHO and UNICEF with the aim of reducing infant mortality and morbidity by providing comprehensive care (curative, preventive and promotional) for the problems of sick children in health facilities.

b. Procedure or methodology

The following procedures are used in the application of this programme:
Once the child's identity, care and other details such as weight, temperature, problems or complaints have been completed, the health worker examining the child will ask questions or observe the following:

a) **Look for general signs in the child**:

1) Any unconscious or lethargic child
2) Any child with a history of convulsions
3) Any child who does not suck, drink or eat
4) Any child who vomits everything they eat.
5) Any child who has convulsions

The presence of one of the signs obliges :

- A referral to the hospital if you are at the health centre
- Compulsory hospitalisation if in hospital.

b) Look for the child's main symptoms.

This is to assess and classify symptoms in terms of their severity and associated signs.
These signs are :

- **Cough or difficulty breathing.** If this sign is present, the respiratory movements and signs such as wheezing, stridor and wheezing should be counted and the cough classified. It may be **severe pneumonia** if there are danger signs such as stridor, wheezing or wheezing, or simple pneumonia if the cough is accompanied by rapid breathing, greater than 40 movements per minute for a child over 1 month old and 50 movements for a child under 1 month old. In this case, hospitalisation is essential.

- **Looking for diarrhoea**

Ask for how long? And if there is blood in the stools, then classify the diarrhoea according to dehydration (level or degree) and duration (persistent diarrhoea lasting more than 14 days) or according to the presence of blood (dysentery).

- **Look for fever** (or history of fever) and then look for associated signs such as stiff neck, signs of measles and signs of danger as seen previously.
  A fever can therefore be classified as: a very serious febrile illness, if the neck is stiff, which is a danger sign. Malaria if there is only fever. Severe or complicated measles if there is a KOPLICK sign.
- **Search for an ear problem (ENT):**

a) Pus discharge (purulent otitis)
b) Pain on pressure in the tragus or behind the ear, which can be classified as acute ear otitis, chronic ear infection if more than 14 days and mastoiditis if there is swelling behind the ear.

- **Check for anaemia** :

By palmar pallor and classify as severe anaemia according to the pallor. See also Hb dosage

- **Look for signs of malnutrition.**

➢ By losing weight
➢ By oedema
➢ By weight/age ratios and classify as chronic or moderate acute MEP.

- **Look for signs of probable symptomatic HIV infection**

- Growth problems
- Tuberculosis in children
- Adenopathy in the neck or axillae
- Parotid swelling
- Dental problems
- Prolonged fever
- Chronic diarrhoea, etc.

- **Request vaccines: (EPI)**

Refer to the vaccination calendar to find out which vaccinations your child has received and check for any delays.

- **Ask about Vit A supplementation**

Give vitamin A if the child is behind schedule or has not received it for 6 months. It is given from 6 months to 5 years.

Finally, once all these problems have been assessed and classified, the child will be treated according to each problem and then transferred or given an appointment for a follow-up visit.

O.4.SOME BACKGROUND INFORMATION

Childhood illnesses in the tropics (intertropical region) are generally preventable.

Of these, around ten are genuine, the most frequently encountered:

- Malaria;
- Respiratory infections;
- Infantile diarrhoea, especially diarrhoea in early-weaned children;
- Protein Energy Malnutrition (PEM)
- Some infectious diseases: measles, tetanus, etc.
- Worm diseases
- TBC ;
- Poisoning, especially from indigenous medicines
- Sickle cell disease
- Bilharzia (in the case of HIV/AIDS as an opportunistic disease)

The general cause of infant mortality is a correlation with the causes linked to hygienic, educational and other factors listed below:

1) **Causes of prenatal mortality**. They are due to the mother's poor health during birth, which is the cause of foetal MEP, i.e. foetal infection leading to death in utero.
2) **Maternal and neonatal causes (from birth to 28 days).** These are due to the delivery by incompetent personnel, who are responsible for mortality:
    - By dystocia, by trauma.
    - Infection (neonatal septicaemia, umbilical infection) tetanus, anaemia due to careless cord ligation.
3) **Postnatal causes (from 1 to 12 months)**

They are due :

- gastroenteritis
- respiratory infections

Gastroenteritis is the result of an infection associated with dirty water (contaminated water, presence of flies, absence of latrines, ignorance on the part of the mother).

4) **Causes of death in children aged 1 to 5 or pre-school age.**

They are due :

- The MEP
- Measles
- Enteritis ;
- Malaria
- Intestinal worms
- TBC
- Anaemia
- Accidents

5) **Causes of death in school-age children** (6 to 12 years): These are due to the causes listed above, but mainly : -MEP -Verminosis -Malaria -Infectious diseases -Skin diseases
   In view of the above, each nurse must master the organisation of any activity aimed at prevention, including the activities carried out at the CPS.

O.5.ORGANISATION OF THE CPS

- Registration

It records everything that could affect the health of the child or mother, as well as any medical history. Registrations made at each CPS must be collated in order to compile activity statistics. This involves keeping a register.

- **Weighing and measuring**

The scales will be used once a month, and the child's weight must be taken regularly each month in order to monitor his or her weight development, not forgetting his or her height (cfr health pathway). The nurse must know the relationship between weight and age.

- **Clinical examination of the child and recommendations**

The examination is the most important moment when we try to take stock of a health situation.
It consists of :

- Listen to the mother's complaints or questions
- Observe the child and mother, drawing attention to risk factors.

If the mother does not report any difficulties, a full history and clinical examination are required.
Once the diagnosis has been made, the decision has to be taken. Interpreting the weight curve is very important.
In principle, the curve should be rising, not stationary, let alone falling.

- **Vaccinations**

We base ourselves on the EPI vaccination calendar that all nurses are required to know (see paediatrics course).

- **Administering medicines**

Medicines can be administered if necessary, but mainly vitamin A. If the child requires curative treatment, he or she should be transferred to the curative consultation.

- **Health and nutrition education (CCC)**

It is given at each of the previous stages, and each CPS player (IT, trainee community health nurse, nursing assistant) must be a health educator.

A few concepts relating to the paediatric department

a) Definition

Paediatrics is a special science of medicine that deals with human beings in the process of growth and development, which makes it a complex science. It therefore includes child care (monitoring the child's development), promoting the health of normal children, preventing illness and diagnosing and treating sick children. By convention, paediatrics deals with children from conception to the age of 15.

b) The importance of paediatrics

It's a branch of medicine that everyone has to go through. It is one of the areas in which developing countries lag behind industrialised countries.

Paediatrics remains a speciality in its own right because of the size of the population it envelops (it accounts for 40% of the total population) and the range of disciplines it covers (see course content).

c) Aim of paediatrics

It aims to help children regain their health, prevent illness and help them become adults through health education sessions.

Paediatrics uses the following methods to achieve this:

- The prevention of various infectious diseases through vaccination,
- Early management of childhood illnesses,
- Monitoring of children's growth and development by the CPS,
- Nutritional promotion: encouraging exclusive breastfeeding and food diversification beyond the age of 6 months.

d) Characteristics of paediatric care

1) Paediatric care requires team spirit. This team is made up of: paediatrician, nurses, the child, the mother (the family), etc.
2) Paediatric care must be individualised and adapted to each child's age.
3) This care must promote the child's physical and mental development according to his or her needs,
4) Care techniques must be carried out with particular gentleness, speed and accuracy.

0. The role of the paediatric nurse

The nurse's role with the child in hospital: the nurse is part of a care team. They work in collaboration with the doctor, nursing colleagues, nursery assistants or aids. The nurse's role with a sick child is always part of that team, and can be summed up as follows:

a) Welcoming parents and children ;
b) Making the diagnosis and monitoring the child ;
c) Administering care
d) Harmonising relations between children and their parents.

- **Role in reception**

a) Emergency reception (triage service)

- Nurses need to know how to distinguish a seriously ill child from others
- Excellent technical skills to perform resuscitation quickly and effectively;
- Welcoming and reassuring the family;
- Participating in the doctor's clinical examination,
- Referring the child and his/her parents according to the decisions taken
- Maintaining, replacing and managing care equipment on the ward.

b) Welcoming in the care unit (paediatrics department)

- Welcoming children and their parents.

- Explain how the service is organised.
- Find out the reason for the child's hospitalisation and any para-clinical examinations, and carry them out or have them carried out;
- Carry out the routine procedures involved in any hospitalisation (weighing, height measurements, routine examinations, compiling patient records)

- **The nurse's role in diagnosing and monitoring the child.**

These two roles are inseparable.

The nurse helps to establish the diagnosis by noticing and reporting a new development in the child to the doctor.

Surveillance covers :

- The child's behaviour;
- The state of consciousness
- Assessing the child's appearance

Regardless of the type of surveillance, you must :

- Sufficient staff to carry out the work (3 to 5 beds for an A3, 6 to 10 beds for an A2, 10 to 25 beds for an A1);
- That this surveillance is carried out 24 hours a day (keeping the care plan sheet is essential);
- The appearance of any anomaly in the parameters measured is immediately reported on the monitoring form or the care form.

- **The nurse's role in administering care.**

a) It obeys precise rules that must be respected when administering medicines, because all medicines are potentially dangerous.

What are these rules?

There are 5 just ones:

1) The right medicine
2) The right dose
3) The right route of administration
4) The right time and expiry date
5) Just sick

b) Only medicines prescribed by qualified personnel should be given;
c) Nurses need to know the dosage of the medicines they usually use to avoid prescription errors.
d) The administration of medicines cannot be delegated to auxiliary staff;
e) Whenever a prescription appears obscure, unusual or difficult to carry out, the nurse must ask for explanations or assistance.
f) Control and avoid errors by default or excess when administering medication. Knowledge of the formula for calculating the dose to be administered is essential. The formula is as follows:

$$\boldsymbol{Dose\ demand\acute{e}e} = \frac{\boldsymbol{dose\ \grave{a}\ administrer\ X\ dilution}}{\boldsymbol{concentration}}$$

Once the medicines have been given, make a note on the cardex sheet (name of medicine, time, route, dose, name of carer, any special observations);

g) The times of administration must be respected, depending on the properties of the drugs (half-life).

Other care :

- ➢ They require knowledge of a wide range of techniques, mainly in paediatrics: venous or peripheral infusions (use of G22, G21, G20 etc.) can facilitate venous function in this department.
- ➢ Parenteral injections and umbilical catheterisation.
- ➢ Various treatments such as pharyngeal and digestive aspirations, and humidification during oxygen therapy.

- **The role of the nurse in the relationship with the child and his/her parents**

- ❖ It is the nurse who carries out most of the care;
- ❖ They ensure that the child's comfort and care are not provided by auxiliary staff,
- ❖ He is the one who explains to the child what we want to do with him.
- ❖ It provides parents with information on how to care for their children
- ❖ On discharge, he will provide the necessary explanations about the treatment, the diet to be followed and any homework required.

A few precautions to take during paediatric examinations

1) Do not undress the child directly, but ask the parent to do so;
2) Before auscultating, palpate and warm the hands of the stethoscope or other equipment to be used.
3) Knowing how to distinguish between attitudes to adopt with children aged 1 to 3, 4 to 6, 7 to 9 and 10 to 15.
4) Assess the child's vital signs and consciousness (height, temperature, heart rate, heart rate, weight, etc.).
5) Know how to examine the child's skin, eyes, vision, ears, abdomen, etc.
6) Take a good look at the genitals.

1. **Practical organisation of paediatric activities. The nurse's role in the paediatric department is vital.**

Here are the main points to follow:

- Ensuring a good reception (knowing how to distinguish the child's state of seriousness before compiling the file);
- Providing initial nursing care (venous access, correct positioning, hygiene care, laboratory tests, etc.).
- Call in the doctor and present the case, taking into account all the elements of the presentation:
    - Patient identity
    - Main complaints
    - Presumptive ruling
    - Date of arrival
    - Condition on arrival
    - Care already administered
- Carry out medical prescriptions and recommendations

- Monitoring the child's condition and identifying any disturbed needs. This involves a detailed interview with the parents
- On discharge, provide health education to the parents, informing them of the pathology at home and how to prevent the illness in the future, and arrange an appointment.

0.6. NOTIONS OF PAEDIATRIC CARE

Paediatrics is a special field of medicine that looks after children from birth to the age of 15.

Note that: a child's growth and development go through the following major stages:

- The embryonic or ante-natal period
- The natal period or childbirth stage
- The post-natal period

1) **The ante-natal period**: is subdivided into two sub-periods:

a) The embryonic period: this covers the 1er trimester of pregnancy.

b) The foetal period: this covers the 2e and 3e trimesters of pregnancy.

2) **The birth period.** It starts at the beginning of the W. of childbirth until the umbilical cord is cut.

This period lasts 12 hours in multiparous women and 15 hours in primiparous women. This is the shortest period in the growth and development of the individual. This period requires close monitoring, as any prolonged W. leads to foetal distress, with the risk of perinatal death or serious neurological sequelae.

Attention

We must remember that thousands of children die every day during this period.

3) **The post-natal period**

This is the longest period in a child's growth and development. This period runs from the moment the umbilical cord is cut to the post-pubertal period.

The post-natal period includes the following sub-periods:

a) **The earliest period**: the first 24 hours of the newborn's life
This period remains the most dangerous, as 50% of neonatal deaths occur during this period.

b) **The early period**: this is represented by the 1ère week. This is a very important period that needs to be monitored, as ¾ of deaths occur during the 1ère week of a newborn's life.

c) **The late neonatal period**: from day 8e to day 28 .e

d) **The infant period**: from 2e months to 2 years. This period is characterised by very accelerated growth and development, with the child doubling its weight between 3e and 5e months of age, tripling its birth weight at 1 year and quadrupling its weight at 2 years. This is an important period, during which the child is exposed to a number of infectious diseases, making it essential to prevent them through vaccination.

e) **The school period**: from the age of 7 to 12, a period characterised by major intellectual, spiritual and psychological acquisitions.

f) **Puberty**: from the age of 12 to 15. This is a period of transition between childhood and adulthood.

g) **Adolescence:** from 15 years onwards.

4) **Administration of paediatric care**

- **A few basic principles.**

➢ Paediatric care requires a team approach (doctor, nurse, child, family),

➢ Paediatric care must be adapted to each child and his or her age;

➢ Paediatric care must be carried out gently, quickly and accurately. This must be done through doses that must be well calculated.

- **Administering medicines**

For medicines in tablet form, you need to look at the strength of each tablet and see the portion corresponding to the prescribed dose.

Medicines should always be prescribed in mg and not in terms of tablets. It is the person administering the medicine who must translate the dose into the number of tablets.

EX: 1) You have been prescribed 125mg of paracetamol. If you have a 500mg tablet corresponding to 125mg/500mg=1/4 tablet

2) You have been prescribed 250mg of paracetamol. If you have 500mg, 250mg corresponds to 250mg/500mg=1/2co

➢ **For liquid medicines (oral or injectable)**; the prescribed dose must be translated into the volume of liquid medicine to be administered according to the formula :

$$\textbf{Volume de médicament liquide à administrer} = \textbf{dose prescrite (en mg par ex.)X dilution/concentration}$$

Tapez une équation ici.

Example:

We prescribed 200 mg of paracetamol syrup to reduce the fever. The bottle reads:

Paracetamol syrup 1 20 mg /5ml

Prescribed dose=200 mg.

Dilution=5ml.

Concentration=120mg for 5ml.

Volume of paracetamol to be administered=200mgx5ml/120mg=8.3ml syrup.

You want to administer ampicillin 230mg IV to a child. You have a 500mg vial of ampicillin which you dilute to 5ml. How many ml of ampicillin should you give the child?

$$Qté\ d'ampi\ à\ donner = 230mgX\ 5/500mg = 2{,}3ml.$$

Genta prescribes a child 20mg 2ml/80mg=0.5ml.

NB: For some very small doses, it is difficult to draw them up in the usual syringes (2cc, 5cc). EX.0, 04 ml.

In this case, it is advisable to dilute a certain amount of the product beforehand.

You want to give 5mg of Gentamycin, you have an ampoule of 80mg/2ml. number of ml to give=5mg X 2ml/80mg=0.12ml difficult to aspirate. First you need to take 9ml of distilled water and add it to 1ml/40mg of Gentamycin. This will give 10ml/40mg. Then calculate 5mgX10/40mg =1.2ml

For infusions, precision means calculating the flow rate, so that the prescribed liquid can be administered over a specific period.

The calculation of the infusion rate and even the transfusion rate follows the following procedure:

$Nombre\ des\ gouttes\ \grave{a}\ faire\ couler\ par\ minute =$

$Nombre\ de\ gouttes\ au\ volume\ de\ liquide\ \grave{a}\ donner./\ temps\ en\ minutes.$

NB: To find the number of drops corresponding to the volume of liquid, simply multiply the quantity by 20 if you are using a macro-drop infusor (1ml=20 drops) or by 60 if you are using a micro-drop infusor (1ml=60 drops).

To get the time in minutes, multiply the number of hours required to run the infusion by 60 minutes.

You want to administer 200ml in 4 hours.

Macro drop kit: 200ml 20/4 60 minutes=4000/240=16.6 drops/min. i.e. 17 drops. Or **else** $\boldsymbol{quantit\acute{e}\ de\ liquide\ en\ ml/\ temps\ en\ heures\ x3}$.

= 200/4x3=200/12=16.6 drops or 17 drops/min?

a) Micro-dropper kit: 200 mlX60/4x60 min= 1200/240= 50 drops. Or $\frac{\boldsymbol{Qt\acute{e}\ de\ liquide\ \ en\ ml}}{\boldsymbol{Nbre\ d'heures}}$.

CHAP.I NEONATAL NURSING CARE

Neonatology is a branch of paediatrics that cares for children from birth to 28 days (maximum 30 days).

The development of antenatal diagnosis and improvements in the monitoring of high-risk pregnancies mean that neonatology is working more and more closely with the obstetric team to provide better care for the newborn in the labour ward. This has led to the creation of a new science, perinatology, which includes neonatology, obstetrics, developmental biology, genetics and foetology.

I.1. A FEW DEFINITIONS

- The perinatal period: is the period from 22 S.A. to 7 days after birth.
- The neonatal period: is the period between birth and the 28ᵉ day of extra-uterine life. This period is subdivided into 3 :

❖ Very early neonatal period: from birth to 24 hours of life.

❖ Early neonatal period: from 1ᵉʳ to 7 days of age.

❖ Late neonatal period: from 8ᵉ days to 28ᵉ days of life.

N.B.: Full-term babies are those born between 37ᵉ and 42ᵉ S.A.

Premature birth being between 22 and 37SA

1. The role of the nurse: birth care (in the delivery room).

Care in the 1ères minutes following birth must follow a certain order and must take place within the first 5 minutes. These are :

a) Airway clearance

Directly in the post-expulsion room, the midwife holds the baby's legs, head down, to help clear the airways by drainage. The cord can be tied to continue clearing the airway on the treatment table in the delivery room.

The mouth and pharynx are cleaned using a finger covered with a sterile compress, and the mucus in the mouth, pharynx and nose is suctioned out using a bulb or respirator.

During this suction manoeuvre, the child should be in the **Trendelemburg** position, with the head deflected by a small cushion over the shoulder blades.

b) Establishing the APGAR score.

This is not care in the strict sense of the word, but the first examination that guides the action to be taken. This consists of examining the child using a number of criteria to assess the vitality of the newborn.

1) Skin appearance or colour
2) Pulse
3) Grimace (reaction to stimuli)
4) Activities (muscle tone).
5) Breathing

Each criterion is given a score ranging from 0 to 2 points, depending on the state of the n.

Parameters	Quotation		
	0 point1 point	**1 point**	**2 points**
Skin appearance	Generalized cyanosis	Pink with cyanotic tips	Rose or skin erythrosis
Pulse (heart rate).	Nil or $<$ 60 beats/min	60 to 100 beats/min	$>$ 100 beats/min
Grimace (reaction to stimuli)	None	Weak reaction	Lively reactions (lively movements).
Muscular activity	Null (child is flaccid)	Extremity bending	Active movements, forced flexion of limbs
Breathing	None	Slow, irregular (weak cry)	Regular (vigorouscry)

Normally the **APGAR** score is good, between 7 and 10/10.
Between 4 and 6: **moderate asphyxia:** in this case the child must be resuscitated. The prognosis here is good.
If the score is $\leq$ 3/10 this is **severe asphyxia** or **white asphyxia**. In this case the child is said to be in a state of apparent death.
The APGAR score is assessed at 1ère , 5ème and 10ème minutes.

c) Cord care

After expulsion, the midwife places 2 kocher thimbles on the cardoon 10cm from the umbilicus, these 2 thimbles being separated from each other by 2cm, then she cuts the centre of 2 thimbles using a pair of scissors. He finishes by tying a double knot of sterile cotton thread (an umbilical string) 3cm from the umbilicus: tie a simple circular knot, tie a knot and finally fold over the stump and dress with an antiseptic (denatured alcohol, iodine, povidone, etc.).

d) Skin care

This consists of wiping mucus, mucus and blood from the skin (drying the child); but leaving the vernix caseosa in place, which conveys heat to the skin and protects it from the cold.

e) Eye care or CREDE.

This involves instilling eye drops into the child's eyes to prevent ophthalmia or gonococcal conjunctivitis in newborns.

Tetracycline 1% ophthalmic ointment is usually used: a 1 cm strip in each eye as soon as possible, preferably within an hour of birth.

f) Examining the newborn

a) Inspection of the child.
b) Measurements

c) Look for malformations: harelip, feet, bots, anal imperforation, etc.
d) Note the child's sex

g) **Dress and cover the newborn (hat, linen, etc.)**
h) **Identify the newborn** (place a bracelet with the child's name or the mother's name, sex and date of birth on it).
i) **Systematic prophylaxis of haemorrhagic disease of the newborn.**

Vit K is necessary for the blood coagulation process. Newborn babies are born with low levels of Vit K, which exposes them to the risk of newborn haemorrhagic disease. As a preventive measure, Vit K is therefore systematically administered to every newborn at birth. Infants under 3 months of age who have not received their Vit K injection should receive it as soon as possible.

Vit K is administered intramuscularly (IM). Use the smallest needle diameter possible: if$26G \geq 2500gr,\ 23G < 2500gr$. If the newborn has a venous line in place (for another reason), Vit K can be administered intravenously (IV).

NB: once opened, phytomenadione ampoules must be used immediately or thrown away.

Dosage and administration

Phytomenadione (Vit K1): IM injection into the anterolateral aspect of the thigh during the first few hours of life.

- $\geq 1500gr: 1ml$ administered as a single dose (= 0.1ml of the 2mg/0.2ml solution).
- $< 1500gr: 0{,}5mg$ administered as a single dose (=0.05ml of the 2mg/0.2ml solution).

Vit K1 can also be taken orally

I.2. THE ROLE OF THE NURSE IN NEONATAL RESUSCITATION.

It should be stressed that asphyxiated newborns are very fragile and tired, as all their energy is consumed in initiating respiratory movements.

A great deal of pain and comfort is therefore required when resuscitating a suffering newborn, as any sudden action causes additional stress for the newborn.

Treatment is based on observing the "ABC D" rules of resuscitation, according to the following principles:

A: Air ways: i.e. freeing the airways

B: Breathing: This is the supply of oxygen, which is the essential element in the resuscitation of an infant in distress.

This will prevent the onset of sequelae, especially neurological ones. Oxygen can be supplied using an Ambu bag, an oxygen concentrator (oxygenator) or an oxygen cylinder...

C: Circulation: The aim is to maintain good blood circulation by performing external cardiac massage. Once ventilation has started, the newborn does not always breathe, the heart rate must be assessed. If it is < 60btt/min, start cardiac massage.

The most effective method is to use two thrusts on the lower third of the sternum, with both palms and fingers encircling the chest. The respective rhythms of compressions and ventilation are 90 compressions for 30 insufflations per minute (i.e. 3 cardiac compressions for one insufflation). The combination of ventilation and external cardiac massage ideally requires two people to perform it effectively, unless the intubation tube is already connected to the delivery room ventilator. ECM is stopped as soon as the spontaneous heart rate is above 60btt/min.

D: DRUGS (Medicines): this is the last element of resuscitation and is optional.

It consists of using a number of resuscitation drugs, in particular :

- ✓ BINA: 1-2ml/Kg IVD diluted administered to combat acidosis.
- ✓ Hypertonic glucose serum 50% 1-2ml/Kg IVDL followed by SG 10% 80 to 100ml/Kg in which we add Ca^{++} (Calcium gluconate) 0.4ml/Kg + AZANTAC 5ml/Kg to run for 24 hours to compensate for the energy loss observed in the event of asphyxia.
- ✓ CAFFEINE: a bronchial dilator, 5mg/Kg IVDL is given.
- ✓ DIAZEPAM: 0.5mg/Kg or PHENOBARBITAL 5mg/Kg to be prescribed in the event of convulsions in newborns indicating anoxic encephalopathy.
- ✓ ADRENALINE: 0.05mg to 0.03mg/Kg IVD as a cardiac stimulant indicated in cases of bradycardia.

NB: resuscitation of the newborn should not exceed 20 to 25 minutes. After this time, resuscitation should be discontinued and the neonate given a maintenance infusion.

Good resuscitation requires at least 3 or 4 people under the supervision of a co-ordinator who assigns specific roles to each person.

Never hit or stimulate the baby repeatedly.

I.3. REARING PREMATURE BABIES.

According to the WHO, a premature baby is any newborn before the age of 37^{e} but with at least 22 S.A, whatever the weight but with at least 500gr.

The role of the nurse

From birth, care must focus on 5 chains in the management of premature babies: **the oxygen chain, the heat chain, the asepsis chain, the feeding chain and the information chain**.

In terms of nursing, the nurse's role must be based on 3 fundamental principles:

- Combating the chill
- Adapting your diet to your abilities and needs.
- Fighting infection

A) Combating the chill

Premature babies weighing less than 1800gr should be raised in an incubator. Those with a birth weight of over 1800gr can be raised in a cradle.

The incubator provides heating adapted to the immaturity of the thermoregulatory system and maintains thermal equilibrium. The incubator also provides humidified oxygenation.

Apart from the incubator, other ways of fighting the cold are :

- Keep the room warm: use heat bulbs, avoid opening windows.
- Radiant heat lamp.
- (Garnish) warmly cover the premature baby: clothing, blankets, etc.
- The "Kangaroo" method, which uses skin-to-skin contact between mother and baby to promote natural warming. This method is currently being promoted because it is effective, inexpensive and presents no risk of burns or infection, as is the case with other methods (incubators, radiant heat lamps).

It also strengthens the affectionate relationship between mother and baby. However, it does require the mother and nursing staff to keep a close eye on breathing, as some premature babies can suffer apnoea during the method. This method should therefore be avoided in cases of **serious respiratory problems**: severe respiratory distress, repeated apnoea attacks.

This method consists of :

1) Place the small baby on its mother's chest, between the two breasts, using a baby carrier called a Kangaroo or a loincloth.
2) Cover mother and baby with a jacket or suitable fabric.
3) Cover baby's head with a bonnet and feet with socks.

It has at least five advantages

- Human warmth.
- No risk of infection.
- Encourages feeding (breastfeeding)
- Reinforces mother-child affection.
- The baby is safe.

B) Adapting your diet to your needs and abilities.

The following principles should be borne in mind when selecting the feed:

- Feed the premature baby early (from the first hour) to avoid hypoglycaemia, hypocalcaemia, dehydration, acidosis and hyperbilirubinaemia.
- Feed the premature baby early by gavage when the birth weight is less than 1500g or when there is no coordination between the sucking and swallowing reflexes.
- Split meals: 8 to 12 meals a day because the stomach's capacity is reduced.
- Give breast milk as it is well tolerated and if it is not good to use commercial milk low in fat (as he has a lipase deficiency) and sodium (as his kidneys have difficulty eliminating sodium).

From birth, premature babies may be undernourished by their parents: 10% glucose serum 60ml/kg on day 1er . Start oral feeding at the same time if the baby weighs more than 1.5 kgs.

Amount of rest to be given

If the premature baby weighs more than 1.5kg and is suckling, there is no need to programme. Milk should be given frequently on demand, as in the case of full-term babies (at least every 2 to 3 hours).

If the baby weighs less than 1.5 kgs, it will be fed through a tube, the quantity must be calculated and a certain rhythm must be followed. The quantity will be calculated as follows:

On day 1er : 60ml/kg and add 20ml/kg each day up to 180ml/kg by day 7ème and more. The daily amount will be given in several meals (8 meals). C.à.d.

1er day : 60ml/kg : 2e day : 80ml/kg ;3e day :100ml/kg ;

4ème day: 120ml/kg ;5ème day:140ml/kg ;6ème day:160ml/kg ;7e day and more 180ml/kg.

Example: a premature baby weighing 1500gr will recieve 90ml to be divided into 8 to 12ml per meal if tolerated. The following day, the dose is increased to 80ml/kg, i.e.

120ml per day, giving 12 to 15ml per meal. We will continue to increase according to tolerance until we reach 180ml/kg.
Generally, during the first 24 hours (for babies weighing less than 1500gr), the premature baby will fast and only receive the infusion, as early altered feeding exposes them to enterocolitis (EUN).
NB: For premature babies weighing less than 1250g, do not give anything by mouth for 48 hours: use 10% glucose by IV (80ml/kg on days 1er and 2e).
Start breastfeeding with SNG at 3ème day in 12 meals and increase to 8 times when he has more than 1250gr.pml.

- ❖ Premature babies weighing between 1250 and 1500 grams should be played with for 24 hours, then start on breast milk at 2e day.
- ❖ Always adapt to digestive tolerance by giving just the quantity tolerated and give liquid IV (G10%) or mixed solution: G10% + RL from day 4e at a proportion of 1/5 RL and 4/5 G10%).
- ❖ Before force-feeding, always aspirate the residue and record the quantity on the card.

Mealtimes :

- ➢ For premature babies weighing less than 1250g = 12 meals.
- ➢ Premature babies 1260 gr to 1800 gr = 8 meals
- ➢ Premature babies weighing over 1800g: 8meals (but these babies are able to suckle, so the tube is not necessary unless they are too weak due to illness.

C) The fight against infection

The role of the nurse in preventing infection in premature babies.

As the premature baby is exposed to infections, we must try to prevent them:

- **Asepsis**

- ➢ The incubator must be cleaned and disinfected every fortnight.
- ➢ Premature care units must be cleaned by vacuuming or wiping with a damp cloth.
- ➢ Staff caring for premature babies must wash and disinfect their hands before touching them, and must strictly observe asepsis in all care given.
- ➢ Avoid going in and out of the premature baby's room.

- **Antibiotic therapy**

Indicated for premature babies born after a risk of infection, particularly after :

1. Membrane rupture
2. Prolonged work
3. Notion of maternal infection or fever
4. Tinged or greenish amniotic fluid
5. The concept of resuscitation
6. Late arrival of the premature baby in the blanket
7. Home birth

- **Prognosis for premature babies**

With better care, premature babies develop successfully and grow well (gain weight and grow).
The chances of a premature baby being viable depend on the following factors:

- The degree of prematurity

- Delivery method
- Causes of childbirth
- The quality of care received

Newborn with an infection

Certain neonatal infections should be feared for their seriousness: meningitis, septicaemia, abdominal infections such as necrotising ulcerative colitis.

On the other hand, local infections such as conjunctivitis and umbilical infection, although benign, should not be underestimated, as they can be a gateway to septicaemia. Depending on the time of onset, a neonatal infection may be early (within the first 24 hours after delivery), early (onset before the 7^{e} day of life) or late (onset after the 7^{e} day of life).

The role of the nurse

1) **Looking for signs of neonatal or probable neonatal infection are :**
    - Fever or hypothermia
    - Convulsions
    - Inability to breastfeed
    - Rapid breathing
    - Nose flapping
    - Lethargy or unconsciousness
    - Domed fontanelle
    - Skin-reddening umbilical region
    - Numerous skin tags
    - Abdominal bloating

The presence of one or more of these signs raises the suspicion of a serious infection in newborns

2) **Signs of neonatal infectious risk**

All you have to do at birth is look for risk factors in the history of the disease.

The anamnesis includes antenatal situations that constitute a risk of infection: these are :

- Maternal fever during childbirth.
- Tainted or foul-smelling amniotic fluids.
- Premature rupture of the water sac.
- Prolonged opening of the E.P. greater than 12 hours to 24 hours.
- Foetal suffering.
- Asphyxia at birth (APGAR<7)
- The concept of resuscitation.
- A poor birth condition.

The combination of more than two risk factors is a sign of high neonatal infectious risk. In these situations, the child should be started on antibiotics at birth, without waiting for signs of neonatal infection.

The role of the nurse in P.E.C.

a) **Setting up a treatment**
    - Antibiotic therapy

b) Feeding the child

If the child is not suckling: place an infusion of glucose solution or mixed solution depending on age. Place a stomach tube to feed expressed breast milk.

c) Monitoring :

- vital signs
- Blood glucose
- General condition

d) In case of localised infection :

E.g. umbilical infection, oral infection, conjunctivitis: Local care.

In case of conjunctivitis

- Clean the eye with a sponge soaked in clean water.
- Apply eye drops.

In case of umbilical infection :

Umbilical dressing with povidone.

In case of stomatitis :

- Cleaning the mouth after feeding with a pad soaked in salt or bicarbonated water
- Brush mouth with nystatin or gentian violet

CHAP II. NURSING CARE IN DISEASES OF THE RESPIRATORY SYSTEM.

Case analysis framework.

Need fdtl	Evocative signs	Intervention	Objective	Observation
1. breathe normally	Dyspnoea, coughing, intercostal and supra-sternal tightness, stridor, nasal flaring	Oxygen therapy, Anti-inflammatory (Dexa 4mg IV)	1. Artificial supply of O_2 . 2. Reduce oedema or inflammation	

II.1. INTRODUCTION

Virginie H. classified the need to breathe normally as the 1[er] of all fundamental needs.

Input O_2, Output CO_2 .

Disruption of this requirement is accompanied by changes in the O_2 supply to the body to varying degrees.

This may be anoxaemia, tissue anoxia, hypoxia or hypoxaemia.

These changes can have harmful and sometimes irreversible consequences for the human body, as in the case of cerebral anoxia.

Very often this disturbance is accompanied by the major danger signs often observed in children:

- The flapping of the wings of the nose
- Dyspnoea
- Coughing.

II.2. THE ROLE OF THE NURSE IN THE PREVENTION OF RESPIRATORY DISEASES.

a. Protect children from the cold and damp by dressing appropriately for the climate and temperature variations.
b. Promoting the body's defences. Good nutrition is one of the most important factors in the frequency and severity of respiratory ailments.

Proteins and vitamins are essential here;

- Boost the body's defences through vaccinations, BCG, Ditecoq (you'll need to check the vaccination schedule for children);
- Improving the quality of housing to reduce the risk of transmission of respiratory diseases.

In this case, you will need to :

- Reduce the number of people per room.
- Ventilation and daytime lighting in the bedroom.

All this is possible thanks to the health education provided by the nurse to the parents.

II.3. ACTION TO BE TAKEN ROLE OF THE NURSE IN UPPER RESPIRATORY TRACT DISEASES.

1. The common cold (flu)

Very often viral, we observe :

- ✓ Sneezing;
- ✓ Clear nasal discharge, sometimes purulent;
- ✓ A red throat;
- ✓ A bit of a cough;
- ✓ Sometimes a slight fever.

Care consists of :

- Remove nasal secretions with a cloth (compress)

To prevent them accumulating and causing superinfection, change the compress each time you evacuate.

- If this is not enough and the nose is blocked, instil children's nose drops, in this case physiological saline or a 0.5% ephedrine-based solution, one drop 3x/day in each nostril/3 days.

The action of ephedrine is vasoconstrictive and therefore congestant. However, adult nasal drops should not be used on children.

- Antibiotics are not normally indicated as they have no effect on the virus.

However, there are cases where they are given especially to **malnourished** children with signs of other illnesses, such as the onset of pneumonia.

Learn to protect the mouth and nose when sneezing to avoid transmission by droplets

2. Sinusitis

This is an infection of the sinuses, i.e. the air-filled spaces in the bones of the face that are connected to the nose.

- Or fever ;
- Certain signs of general infections ;
- Stuffy nose with runny nose;
- Well-localised pain in one or more bones of the face (cheek, forehead)
- Headaches

  The nurse will be able to take better care of this child by adopting the following attitude:

Instill the child's nasal drops (Ephedrine 0.5% to unblock the sinuses).

After cleaning the nose or laying the child's head in a hyper-extended position, leave a drop 3 in each nostril for 3 days.

(ATB, Administration of medicines prescribed by the doctor (analgesics, etc.)

Sinusitis can sometimes be prevented by treating a cold as early as possible with nasal drops for children.

3. Epistaxis

This is nose bleeding. Nosebleeds are not uncommon in children. Some have them regularly.

Most often the septum of the nose known as the "KIESSELBACH ZONE". The nose can be compressed to stop the bleeding. The child presents with abundant epistaxis, swallows it and can then cough it up, which frightens the mother.
The nurse will adopt the following attitude:

1. **Reassure mum that it will pass**; look for the cause: it may be :

- Typhoid fever.
- Coagulation disorder.
- Leukaemia.
- Vitamin K deficiency.
- H TA

2. **Initiate specific treatment if possible.**

EX: T3 in hypertension. This is rare in children.
Administration of vit K if coagulopathy with a hepatic problem. Look for complications.
EX: Hb assay if anaemia, hypotension, etc.
Treat complications if necessary (hydration, transfusion, etc.)
Perform haemostasis of the epistaxis using the technique below:

- Local pressure
- Internal compression with 1% adrenaline tempo
- Cautery if recurrence or serious haemorrhage.

NB: Compresses soaked in adrenaline must remain in place for at least 24 hours.
To insert them, you need to use a stylus.
It must be removed after 24 hours. To do this, first instil physiological saline or distilled water, wait 5 minutes and then remove it.

3. Other causes need to be investigated, e.g. coagulation disorders, leukaemia, cirrhosis of the liver, etc.
4. In the event of significant loss, monitor the child for signs of shock and check the Hb the following day.
5. As a preventive measure, his mother applies Vaseline every evening to the nostrils of children who suffer from recurrent epistaxis.

4. Tonsillitis

This is inflammation of the tonsils.
In some cases :

- Fever ;
- Discomfort;
- Vomiting and diarrhoea;
- Dysphagia ;
- A sore throat,
- Refusal to feed or suckle.
- When the throat is examined using a tongue depressor, swelling and redness of the tonsils and surrounding area are seen, sometimes with drops of pus on the surface (white spots);
- The lymph nodes at the corner of the lower jaw are swollen and tender.

Beware of these signs, as they can lead to dramatic complications:

- Tonsil abscess.
- Rheumatic fever ;

- Otitis media.
- Acute glomerulonephritis
- Endocarditis
- RAA is caused by streptococci.

This is all due to the toxin in the microbes.

Faced with this situation, the nurse will adopt the following attitude:

- All cases of strep throat (red, white spot, with fever, lymph nodes, adenitis, etc.) should be given an energetic t3 with ATBs (preferably penicillin for at least 7 days).

Apart from that, some of the causes appear to be viral, and all that is required is symptomatic treatment (aspirin, gargle, dabbing with methylene blue).

When in doubt, don't hesitate to give a course of penicillin, because there are still too many young people whose lives are shortened by repeated bouts of angina, poorly treated and leading to serious complications such as heart disease, AAR and kidney complications.

In the case of chromic angina with severe symptoms occurring several times a year, a tonsillectomy may be considered by a specialist.

5. Laryngitis

The illness follows a cold or simply accompanies measles. The child presents with :

- An obstructive cough.
- A noise on inspiration called stridor or horning, simply because on inspiration the air passes at high speed through a narrowing space;
- Most often, the throat and epiglottis are red, and the condition may worsen, producing intercostal or supra-sternal indrawing on inspiration;
- The child is restless, pale, cyanotic and behaves as if gasping for air.
- There is a mortal danger and intervention is required to relieve the dyspnoea.

The role of the nurse

- Humidify the air to liquefy laryngeal secretions using specialised equipment (aerosol, O concentrator$_2$, oxygen tent, etc.).
- Give oxygen in a tent, by SNG via an ambu-bag. If the O_2 concentrator is used, care must be taken not to give dry oxygen as it is very irritating when passed through a romper (a young child's garment that leaves the arms and legs bare).
- Reduce oedema with corticosteroids (hydro, dexa);
- Antibiotic therapy as prescribed by the doctor.
- Calming the child with Phenergan (promethazine)
- Rehydrate the child; make sure he or she is getting enough fluids and, if necessary, give small amounts of slightly salted or sugared water or SNG or IV fluids;
- In severe cases, tracheal intubation or tracheotomy may be required.

II.4. LOWER RESPIRATORY TRACT INFECTIONS

1. Bronchitis, bronchiolitis and bronchial asthma

The infection can affect the bronchial tubes: this is bronchitis; it can affect the small bronchial tubes: this is capillary bronchiolitis.

Both can cause bronchial obstruction on exhalation, leading to asthmatic bronchitis (bronchial asthma). Bronchitis and bronchial asthma can also be allergic in origin.

The main common sign is coughing.

However :

a) **In case of bronchitis**
   - He may or may not see the fever
   - On auscultation, you can hear the **snoring rales** scattered about

b) **In cases of bronchiolitis,** we observe :
- Difficult rapid breathing (polypnoea), with flapping of the wings of the nose
- On inspiration, there is considerable intercostal and suprasternal draught.
- On auscultation, the sounds are normal but diminished, although scattered **crackling rales** and sometimes sibilant rales can be heard. Warning: the patient is heading towards fatal anoxia if an energetic t^3 is not introduced as a matter of urgency.

c) In bronchial asthma: dyspnoea accompanied by **sibilance is** more common.
   Generally speaking :
- ➢ Determine the severity of the respiratory problem by means of a more detailed examination, and monitor progress closely (F°, nasal flaring, dyspnoea, sibilance, etc.). Fight the cough, which can be soothed with appropriate medication.
- ➢ The air can be humidified with O_2 by nebulisation to reduce dehydration of the mucous membranes and maintain liquid secretions.

a) **In case of simple bronchitis :**
- Calm coughs if excessive;
- Liquefy sputum with appropriate solutions (cough suppressants);
- Monitor the child regularly to recognise complications early.

b) **In the case of bronchiolitis, it is extremely urgent to :**
- ➢ Place the child in a warm atmosphere
- ➢ If dyspnoea is severe,a bronchodilator should be administered (salbutamol aerosol, valid for all ages).
- ➢ If available, give oxygen ;
- ➢ Broad-spectrum antibiotic therapy is recommended (Ampi-Genta combination);
- ➢ If dyspnoea interferes with fluid or food intake, consider parenteral administration, preferably by IVD;
- ➢ Calm the child with phenergan in small doses;
- ➢ Place the child slightly upside down to facilitate postural drainage of secretions.

c) **In cases of bronchial asthma or asthmatic bronchitis**

A distinction must be made between t^3 asthma attacks and t^3 between attacks.
- ➢ The t^3 of asthma attacks

It consists of :

a) Administration of a salbutamol spray ;
b) Calming the child with a phenergan and reassuring the parents;
c) Oxygen can be very necessary in some difficult cases;
d) If the crisis continues, corticosteroids may be indicated;
e) If there is a fever, combat it and give antipyretics;
f) Give TBAs;
g) If there is dehydration, fluids must be given parenterally.

NB: a cough syrup is also indicated when the attack has improved.

2. The t³ between asthma attacks.

Dealing with the cause: if the cause is a repeated infection, think about preventing sore throats and ear infections;

- Very often in cases of allergic asthma, dust and other allergenic factors (such as smoke, cat hair, etc.) should be avoided as far as possible.

In this case, there is a high level of eosinophilia in the blood and worm eggs in the faeces.

In this case, deworming must be carried out;

- Symptomatic treatment may be administered with promethazine syrup.

3. Bronchopneumonia and pneumonia

Lung infection can affect not only the bronchi but also the alveoli: this is bronchopneumonia.

Involvement may be centred on the alveoli of one of the lungs: this is lobar pneumonia.

The microbes most commonly responsible are :

a. Staphylococci for bronchopneumonia;
b. Pneumococcus, haemophilus, pneumonia viruses.

Although the 2 diseases can be distinguished by their signs and possible complications, the t³ is often identical.

However, here are a few signs for the 2 diseases.

- **Bronchopneumonia**

The onset is abrupt and the situation is sometimes serious in children with colds, flu, measles, whooping cough and malnutrition.

Signs of serious infection include

a) High fever ;
b) Elevated pulse ;
c) Sluggishness (prostration or lethargy) ;
d) State of shock ;
e) Acute dyspnoea ;

- **Pneumonia**.

✓ The start is just as abrupt;
✓ Intense depression sets in as quickly as possible;
✓ High fever during the state period.
✓ Rapid dyspneic R° with severe draught;
✓ Auscultation reveals crackling, fine rales and tubal murmurs.

Complications are less serious than in bronchopneumonia, where there is a combination of snoring and crackling on auscultation.

The role of the nurse.

- **In cases of bronchopneumonia**.

a) Draw up as complete a Dg as possible: this consists of giving the child's real situation (circulatory and respiratory problems);

b) The child should be put to rest in a semi-seated position without tight clothing in a well-ventilated room;

c) You need to look after his diet by giving him semi-liquid foods rich in calories and proteins;

d) Check fever regularly;

e) However, most of the treatment at^3 consists of strong antibiotic therapy (Ampi-Genta combination);

f) If dyspnoea is severe, consider cardiac decompensation and give a fast-acting cardiac tonic (digitalis) and humidified oxygen if available;

g) If there is no improvement, a complication should be suspected and an x-ray should be considered.

- **In case of pneumonia**

➢ Specify Dgc ;

➢ TBAs are effective and make up the bulk of t^3 ;

➢ The prognosis is slightly better than for bronchopneumonia.

Preventive measures include

❖ Ensure vaccination against measles, whooping cough and TBC;

❖ Nutritional education: this is the surest way of increasing children's ability to defend themselves against infection.

4. Pleurisy

Young children suffer from 2 types of pleurisy:

✓ Purulent staphylococcal pleurisy

It is a typical complication of pneumonia and bronchopneumonia.

✓ Serous tuberculous pleurisy

It follows a primary tuberculosis infection.

The child has difficulty breathing and complains of side stitching, i.e. lateral thoracic pain.

It can be seen that he breathes less deeply with one side of his chest and coughs frequently.

Dg is based on pleural puncture, where the fluid removed is purulent or serous.

A chest x-ray should be considered.

The role of the nurse

a) In case of purulent pleurisy

➢ Administer TBAs against staphylococci ;

➢ Regular punctures at first, then after every 2 to 3 days, then less frequently.

➢ Relieve pain and control fever with analgesics and antipyretics.

➢ If the effusion does not subside, a pleural drain is placed to provide continuous suction;

- If the dyspnoea becomes too severe, do not hesitate to puncture the pleura immediately to evacuate as much fluid as possible.

b) **In cases of serous pleurisy**.

A cloudy, citrine fluid is very likely to be of tuberculous origin, following a primary infection.

The t^3 is tuberculosis.

I.4.4. foreign bodies in the respiratory and auditory tracts.

Children can sometimes inhale small objects through their nose or mouth while playing or by accident.

Depending on their size and circumference, these foreign bodies can become blocked at different levels, which is why the nurse will adopt the following attitude:

- **Foreign body in the nose**.

They can cause pain and chronic purulent discharge.

A local anaesthetic can be obtained by placing a cotton wool pad soaked in adrenaline lidocaine in the nostrils (a few drops of 1% adrenaline in 5 CC of 1 or 2% lidocaine). If not, a cautious attempt can be made under the otoscope with a small hook or forceps, taking care not to push the foreign body in any further.

- **Foreign bodies in the ear**

These are often small pearls or insects.

The ear then develops a chronic discharge with no tendency to heal.

First, the ear is washed as for earwax, then the body is carefully removed using a small hook.

If the insect is still there, instil a few drops in the ear to kill it and remove it afterwards.

- **Foreign bodies in the larynx**.

If the foreign body becomes blocked at this point, there is a serious problem of inspiratory stridor.

The nurse must place the child's head downwards, hit the thorax and back to force the foreign body out using air pressure. He will then inspect the child's mouth to see if it can be removed with the forceps.

If this is unsuccessful or if there is severe dyspnoea, try another finger or forceps test, or perform a laryngoscopy or tracheostomy.

- **Foreign bodies in the bronchi**

Frequently, the signs are those of pneumonia.

The history sometimes suggests inhalation of a foreign body, acute dyspnoea and then cough.

The above cause should be considered in any pneumonia that is resistant to T^3 of ATBs, in which case Rx or bronchoscopy should be performed.

I.4.5. Pulmonary tuberculosis and other organs

Never forget that a child who has tbc caught it from someone else.

The role of the nurse is crucial when dealing with a primary infection in a child with TBC, and can be summed up in the following 4 points

- **Screening**

We need to find the person who has contaminated the child and check that other children are not contaminated.

In this case, an examination of the family group or the group the child attends is vital. It is not uncommon for all tests to be negative s^{tt} in cases of malnutrition.
A trial treatment will then be started under medical supervision to monitor progress.

- The treatment

Administer the chemotherapy regimen and ensure that it is followed (see diagram of BBT as recommended by action Damien)

- Monitoring

The nurse who takes charge of a child with primary TBC infection has a duty to check :

a) The regular application of t^3
b) Its effectiveness through bacteriological negativation of sputum

- Health education
- The nurse can point out to the parents that the success of the t^3 depends on the success of the child:
- Correct speed;
- Regularity;
- Respecting the time limit.

CHAP III. NURSING CARE FOR DISORDERS OF THE DIGESTIVE TRACT

Most of the conditions covered in this chapter are not pathological entities in their own right, but rather signs and symptoms whose aetiology must be investigated.

III.1. DIARRHOEA

This is the frequent elimination of excessively liquid stools more than three times in 24 hours.

Role of the nurse (6 roles)

1) **Searching for aetiology**

- Taking a history
- Doing the clinical trial
- Look for fever and respiratory signs such as rhinorrhea;
- Inspect the eardrum and pharynx;
- Carry out para-clinical examinations

⇒Blood culture if temperature > 38

⇒Rx of the thorax in the presence of respiratory signs, also do the coproculture.

⇒Check: stool appearance, colour, consistency, odour, presence or absence of mucus in the stool.

⇒Look for other accompanying signs such as anorexia and vomiting, which may require an IV infusion to be started.

2) **Explain and monitor the diet.**

The anti-diarrhoea diet differs according to the child's age.

The nurse can insist and explain to the mother the need for this diet.

a. **Carrot soup**

Method of preparation: 570gr fresh carrots should be boiled in 1 litre after being cut into small pieces. Boil them for 2h40minutes and then put them through the blender.

- Bring the solution down to 1.5l by adding non-carbonated mineral water.
- Add 3gr of salt for 1l or just under a teaspoon for 0.5l, do not add sugar;
- Shake the container of soup before feeding. You can also give the child raw juice or carrot pulp. Do not add sugar as it is a good medium for fermentation.

b. **Cream of rice or rice water**

- ✓ Method of preparation: boil 2gr of rice in 200ml of water for 10min.
- ✓ Blend in a mixer to avoid lumps;
- ✓ Do not add sugar.

3) **Assess the impact of diarrhoea.**

Look for signs of dehydration (clinical signs), quantify weight loss by weighing, as weight loss >30% is cause for concern and bowel movements >8% should lead to a blood ionogram and the need to start a drip; the child's nutritional status should also be assessed. Dehydration in children should be treated as described in the paediatrics course.

4) **The child must be carefully monitored because of the risk of acute dehydration due to associated fever, refusal to eat or vomiting.**

In this case, it may be necessary to discontinue intravenous feeding and the provision of fluids by IV infusion;

⇒monitoring will continue to focus on the frequency of bowel movements and weight, which must be taken 2x/day

A well-rehydrated child should return to normal weight within 4 hours.

⇒Also monitor: diuresis, eyeball, fontanel

All these elements must be noted on a monitoring form which includes not only the balance of entries and exits but also all the other elements mentioned above and the weight.

5) Diet monitoring

Do not prolong the anti-diarrhoea diet excessively for fear of causing constipation. However, he should gradually return to a normal diet, introducing different foods one by one, depending on the child's age.

6) Monitoring developments

Strict hygiene must be observed during hospitalisation. (Isolate the child if cholera is suspected, hygiene of hands and towels, use of personal objects).

In addition to the anti-diarrhoea diet, the medication prescribed for the aetiology of the diarrhoea should be administered.

NB: Rehydration remains the priority in the event of diarrhoea. Some children suffer from chronic diarrhoea that can threaten their lives through dehydration or malnutrition.

Role of the nurse in this case

⇒Rigorous monitoring;

⇒Participate in the aetiological investigation by seeking out and recording clinical examinations that may point towards a diagnosis

⇒Check the application of t^3 .

III.2. STOMATITIS

The nurse's role in stomatitis (5 roles)

1. Thrush is diagnosed by the presence of stomatitis. In practice, it should be noted that debris is easily differentiated from stomatitis because it does not adhere to the mucosa;
2. Look for hygiene faults in the environment or in bottle preparation;
3. Local treatment ;
4. Before each meal, wrap a compress around the end of a finger after carefully washing your hands. Pour an antifungal oral solution (meuthil) onto the compress and rub vigorously over the tongue, cheeks and gingivo-lingual folds. If the above t^3 is not available, perform a 1% methylene blue touch-up;
5. Preventive treatment

Based on strict hygiene in bottle preparation; and ATB treatment, Nystatin oral suspension for 10 days is recommended.

III.3. ANOREXIA.

The role of the nurse.

- To look for parasites, the following lab tests are considered: E.G., stool examination.
- Take care of food hygiene. Ask the mother about the child's eating habits;
- Giving children a taste for food again. The educational aspect comes into play here.
  After treating the cause, give an appetite stimulant such as juice, fruit, vegetables, etc.
- Administer the tranquilliser in cases of anorexia nervosa.

III. 4. VOMITING AND INTESTINAL WORMS IN CHILDREN

A. Vomiting

The role of the nurse

1. Observe vomiting +: appearance and associated signs ;
2. Assess the condition of the skin, liver, spleen and peristalsis;
3. The t^3 will depend on the cause itself.

Steps to take during vomiting :

- Aspirate the V^O + to facilitate breathing.
- Carrying out lab tests
- Avoid using a bottle with a large teat
- Thicken and split the meal if the child is already eating.
- Allow the child to regurgitate by placing him or her in a prone position.
- Place the child in a safe position (supine position), turning the head to one side.
- In a newborn, the cause must be sought, and a physical examination carried out, looking for an imperforate anus, noting the colour, smell, frequency of V^o + and any associated signs. If the child's condition worsens, L.P. can be performed if the child has meningitis.

B. Intestinal worms

The role of the nurse

a) Educate on hand and environmental hygiene, especially to prevent parasites through health education;
b) Diagnosis by stool sampling and examination,
c) Administer prescribed medication according to cause

III.5. CONSTIPATION

The nurse's role

- ✓ Check the date of the last bowel movement and the presence of intestinal peristalsis,
- ✓ Reassure yourself about the accompanying signs (Stt V^O +);
- ✓ Check your diet;

- ✓ If the constipation is not organic, it can be relieved by small means such as laxatives (honey) and a diet based on fruit and vegetables;
- ✓ Find out about the frequency, consistency and colour of bowel movements.

In principle, a normal child should pass 2 to 3 soft stools.

- ✓ Teach the baby to defecate at specific times that correspond to the mother's available time;
- ✓ Do gymnastics (physical exercise for the child) to stimulate defecation;
- ✓ When the child is fed, encourage regurgitation by placing him on his stomach and patting him a little on the back.

Recommend drinking plenty of water;

- ✓ Stimulate the defecation reflex by inserting the bulb or a small piece of soap into the child's anus.

III.6.THE CHILD WITH A BIG BELLY

This may be due to the accumulation of air from food in the faeces, intestinal obstruction or the accumulation of fluid in the case of ascites, or an increase in the volume of the abdominal organs, liver and splenomegaly.

The role of the nurse

- ❖ Look for the cause and treat it if possible
- ❖ Advisor
- ❖ Perform certain nursing procedures: introduce a rectal suction, an SNG and a bladder suction at the same time to evacuate as much air and faeces as possible, and if possible perform a palliative puncture.

CHAP. IV. NURSING CARE IN CARDIOCIRCULATORY DISEASES

IV.1. HEART FAILURE

The role of the nurse

It has 3 levels

- Diagnosing the disease
- Introducing t3
- Ensuring surveillance

a) diagnose the disease

The diagnosis of this disease is based on :

- Decubitus dyspnoea
- Painful hepatomegaly

. Tachycardia >140 btt/m but radiological sign: cardiomegaly

b) Introducing t^3

1) Cardiac tone (generally digoxin)

It is a dangerous drug because the therapeutic dose is close to the toxic dose.

Its toxicity is manifested by heart rhythm disorders. The pulse must therefore be counted before each dose is taken or administered.

- If bradycardia is observed < at 80 btt/min
- An irregular rhythm or the appearance of tachycardia > at 200btt/min dioxin should not be administered in this case an ECG should be performed as a matter of urgency.

2) T^3 based on diuretics

- Furosemide lassis causes urinary leakage of K, which can be dangerous and must be systematically compensated for by eating bananas.
- Diuresis should be monitored
- Weight gain 2 times a day morning and evening

3) Salt-free diet: is essential for t3.

It is necessary to check that this is strictly applied and to explain the procedure to parents before they leave hospital.

4) Water restriction

If necessary, the start of the infusion must not exceed 50ml/kg/day.

5) Position: put the patient in a semi-seated position.

c) **Monitoring**: There are two types of monitoring: clinical and ECG.

Surveillance element.

- HR: should be checked by cardiac auscultation and not by palpation of the peripheral pulse. It should be measured at rest, at best during sleep.
- FR: skin colouration - weight, which must be taken 2x/day, - diuresis using a Foley catheter n°4, 6, 8, 12, paediatric n°.

ECG monitoring

Other nursing care for cardiac I.

They consist of :

- Antibiotic therapy for respiratory infections.
- Oxygen therapy

- Respiratory physiotherapy ;
- Feeding by force-feeding, if necessary with Nélaton soda.

CHAP.V. NURSING CARE IN DISEASES OF THE NERVOUS SYSTEM

V.1. MENINGITIS

The role of the nurse

1) **Diagnosis of the disease**: the diagnosis of meningococcal meningitis is based on L.P., the technique of which must be well understood in paediatrics.

As soon as the L.P. has been taken, the sample is immediately taken to the lab, sealing the jar tightly.

2) **Administration of medicines**

➢ The t^3 is based on the administration of an IV solution (SG 50%+RL)

The amount of serum to be infused is 50 to 60ml/Kg/day. The infusion can then be reduced when the child starts to eat.

P.O. feeding must be stopped on Day 1er as long as the child is vomiting and there are problems with consciousness, which may be the cause of false swallowing.

The t^3 ATB is started immediately after P.L. as soon as any louche or purulent fluid is observed.

➢ Adjuvant therapeutic measures can also be applied during the first 3 or 4 days and consist of :
    - Stop the convulsion.
    - Fighting fever.
    - Convulsion prevention consists of administering diazepam every 4 hours instead of using phenobarbital because it has a delayed effect.
    - Treatment of fever :
        - Undressing the child
        - Wet wrap
        - Administer Pct and/or ASA if possible

3) **Monitoring the child**

Goal :

✓ Assess the t^3 and its effectiveness in order to detect any complications.

✓ The monitoring elements are clinical and biological.

a) **During the first 48 hours.**

Monitor: pulse, breathing, temperature, state of consciousness by measuring the PC every day;

PL carried out after 48 hours at temperature to check sterilisation of the CLR

b) **In the days that follow and in the absence of complications.**

- It is necessary to take a daily t^3 ;
- A P.L. is issued before the t^3 is stopped.
- The effectiveness of t^3 is judged by :

- Fever reduced and normalised;
- Disappearance of consciousness after 48-72 hours;
- Slow regression of meningeal signs.
- The effectiveness of t^3 is confirmed by the sterilisation of the CSF.

As soon as the child is no longer conscious, he or she can be fed by mouth and the infusion reduced. t^3 is stopped 10 to 15 days after the L.P.

4) Screening for complications.

Expect complications:

- If F° or consciousness disorders persist after 72 hours of t^3 ;
- If convulsions or neurological signs (cranial nerve paralysis) occur;
- If neurovegetative disorders are observed, such as changes in pulse, temperature and respiratory rate, and particularly in infants, vo+, bulging fontanelle or rapid increase in head circumference.

The appearance of any of these signs must be reported so that the necessary measures can be taken quickly:

- ✓ Look for a focus outside the meninges;
- ✓ P.L. to check resistance to ATB ;
- ✓ Ophthalmological examination (F.O.) ;
- ✓ ECG.

Even in the absence of complications, in the acute period the search for sequelae must be systematically carried out before discharge from hospital by the following measures:

- ➢ A careful clinical and neurological examination;
- ➢ An audiogram
- ➢ An F.O

As long as the child is febrile and the CSF is not sterile, hygiene measures must be applied.

V. 2. CONVULSIONS

The role of the nurse

- ❖ **Knowing how to diagnose a convulsion :**
- ➢ By observing abnormal movements, the topography and type of which are noted;
- ➢ Loss of consciousness confirmed by non-response to stimuli

EX: nipple pinch.

- ❖ In all cases, the time and duration of the attack are noted.
  Remains to be asked consist of :
- ✚ Undressing the child;
- ✚ Aspirate naso-bucco-pharyngeal secretions;
- ✚ Oxygenating the child ;
- ✚ In the event of a tonic seizure with a risk of biting the tongue, fit a solid mayo cannula attached to allow secretions to be correctly aspirated.

In the event of a prolonged seizure, respiratory depressant drugs may be administered or the child intubated;

- ✚ Apply valium or phenol to stop convulsions
  Carefully note the time of injection if it is valium. If possible, ventilate the child by mask.
- ✚ If the seizure has not been stopped after 15 minutes, resume diazepam and double the dose;

- Urgent systematic etiological research
- To take the temperature, make a curve;
- Have blood glucose and blood calcium levels tested as a matter of urgency;
- Make the L.P. specifying the pressure, the aspect, the elements (G.R, GB, Protein);
- Perform antibiogram culture ;
- Administration of other medicines prescribed by the doctor.

5) Other treatments: strong antibiotic therapy (Ampi+Genta)

CHAP.VI. TREATMENT OF BLOOD DISEASES

VI.1. ANAEMIA

The role of the nurse

a) If the anaemia is severe (in relation to the signs of severity) paleness of the mucous membranes and teguments, cyanosis, polypnoea, asthenia, fluttering of the wings of the nose, jaundice and from a para-clinical point of view ; (Hb < 5g/%) the nurse may :

❖ Consider transfusing compatible blood, iso group if HIV negative. The following precautions must be taken during transfusion:
  - Donate blood that is fresh or that has been stored in the fridge for no more than 21 days after collection;
  - Do not expose the blood to the sun if cold, keep in the fridge;
  - Do not shake the Baxter containing the blood very hard;
  - Take into account the flow rate during the transfusion: It will be slow at the beginning and gradually increase until it reaches 4 g/Kg/minute;
  - The quantity of blood to be transfused will depend on the t^x of Hb. The formula to be used to calculate the total quantity is : $5XP(15 - Hb)$

In practice, the amount of blood to be received per child should not exceed 20 CC/Kg/Days.

For premature babies it is 10CC/Kg/Days.

- During the transfusion, the nurse must remain at the patient's side for the first 15 minutes to monitor any possible reactions by keeping an eye on the pulse, the temperature and the patient's general condition (face);

b) If moderate anaemia

- Look for the cause in the history (ask about the diet) and a recent infection;
- On clinical examination, look for pallor, jaundice, oedema, cardiac decompensation, splenomegaly, polypnoea;
- Lab tests: Hb, Emel test, G.E. and fresh stools;
- If no cause is identified, repeat stool tests for hookworms; give iron orally and protein for 1 month.

VI.2. SICKLE CELL ANAEMIA.

The role of the nurse

a) Prevention:

- ✓ Regular use of a vasodilator (Hidergine) in preventive doses. This treatment can be administered continuously or discontinuously;
- ✓ Preventive correlation of anaemia by :
- ▪ Balanced diet rich in protein and minerals.
- ▪ Folic acid supplement for long periods.

NB: long-term treatment with iron is contraindicated as there is a risk of it accumulating in the liver and heart.

- ✓ Chemoprophylaxis of malaria: prevention of hookworm infection

- ✓ A healthy lifestyle to prevent infections (vaccinations, appropriate clothing, wound care and early consultations);
- ✓ An oral Ca supplement would be useful;
- ✓ It would be advisable to set up a special monitoring service for children with sickle cell disease within our health facilities, either during pre-school consultations;
- ✓ Parents will be informed about preventive measures and other possible solutions for their future children;
- ✓ Incest is not recommended.

b) On the curative side.

- ➢ In the event of a crisis, curative treatment is often based on transfusion and the administration of vasodilators. Blood transfusion is recommended in cases of severe deglobulation (severe anaemia).
- ➢ Oxygen therapy is also recommended.
- ➢ Vasodilators are given by IV injection or infusion in G5%.

Infusions containing 5% glucose have a favourable effect on capillary circulation through falciformation;

- ➢ Analgesics are used to relieve pain;
- ➢ TCAs against staphylococci are mainly used against osteomyelitis.
- ➢ In the event of shock, corticosteroids can be used;
- ➢ Anti-malarial drugs are always indicated because associated malaria aggravates the disease.

CHAP.VII. TRAUMA IN CHILDREN.

VII.1. THE BURN

When dealing with a child who has suffered a burn, the nurse should adopt the following attitude:

- ➢ Reassure yourself or ask about the cause of the burn;
- ➢ Carry out a general examination of the child and look for signs of shock: rapid, thready or imperceptible pulse.
- ▪ Nose flapping
- ▪ Cooling the extremities
- ▪ Oliguria
- ▪ Look for severe pain if present;
- ➢ Assess the burn according to its condition and depth using the WALLACE rule for paediatrics.
- ▪ Look for signs of infection ;
- ▪ Do the lab test to monitor the Hb level;
- ▪ Take a haematocrit and blood ionogram.

a. Prevention

Simple precautions regarding fire, hot liquids or electricity can simply prevent fatal or disabling burns to children.

The greatest danger is letting children play near food preparation areas when there are no adults to supervise them.

b. Curative.

The first steps to take at home :

- If a child is burnt by a hot liquid or object, the pain can be minimised by immersing the burnt part of the body immediately in clean cold water;
- If several minutes have passed, it is too late, or you can simply cover the burned area with a clean, freshly ironed cloth;
- Relieving pain: severe pain must always be relieved as it can contribute to a state of shock;
- Compensating for lost fluids. A burn is a case of fluid loss for which we must provide the normal fluid intake plus an additional amount of P.O. or IV by calculating as follows:

- Normal intake=150CC/Kg/Jrs.
  Maximum 100ml/Drs before one year and 100CC/Kg/Drs after 1 year.
- Additional intake: add physiological 20ml/Kg/Drs as required for every 10% of body surface area that has been burnt.
- The best parenteral solutions to use are :
  - Haemacèle
  - Plasma substitute.
  - Alternatively Ringer lactate

ORS can be added if the patient is able to drink.

In the case of a burn with signs of shock, the best solution is a haemacel.

- **Local care**

Once the pain has subsided, the entire burned area is washed with lukewarm, soapy water or soap and all dirt and skin debris is removed.

Dressing should preferably be carried out in an operating theatre, where strict asepsis rules apply.

Avoid contact between the wound and lingues.

- **Anti-infection treatment**
    - Administering ATBs ;
    - Prevent tetanus by sero-vaccination (VAT+SAT). If the child has already been vaccinated, have a booster.
    - Anti-malarial t[3] is necessary.

CHAP.VIII: GENERAL INFECTIOUS DISEASES IN CHILDREN.

VIII.1. VIRAL DISEASES

1) Measles

The role of the nurse.

In the case of a child with measles, the nurse's role is to :

a. Isolating the child

Although the contagious period precedes the eruption, hospitalisation should be limited to fragile children or those living in unfavourable conditions, and an IM Gammaglobulin infection is recommended for those around them.

b. Symptomatic treatment

- Prevent dehydration by ensuring adequate fluid intake;
- Disinfect the nose and throat by nasal instillation of physiological saline solution;
- Eye disinfection with argyrol.
- Carry out examinations to detect possible complications such as :
  - ENT to discover an ear infection
  - F.L. to demonstrate hyperleukocytosis;
  - Chest X-ray to detect bronchopneumonia

c. Treatment of complications

- ✓ Otitis: antibiotic-based ear instillation ;
- ✓ Laryngitis: corticosteroids and antibiotics;
- ✓ Oxygen therapy and, if necessary, intubation and artificial ventilation.
- ✓ Neurological complications

Treatment will be aimed at combating convulsions and maintaining viral function.
It will be carried out in the intensive care unit

- ✓ Administration of VAR as a preventive measure

2) Chickenpox

a) Definition

Chickenpox is a highly contagious viral infectious disease affecting children under the age of 5, accompanied by intense itching.

b) Etiology

The causative agent of chickenpox and shingles is the same virus called varicella zoster virus, which belongs to the Herpes virus family. This is a DNA virus: dermoneurotropic, which causes both chickenpox and shingles.

c) Clinical signs

The diagnosis is primarily clinical and evolves in three phases:

1) Incubation phase: lasts 14 days after infectious airborne contact with skin lesions.
2) The invasion phase: this is dominated by fever and adenopathy (axillary lymph nodes, etc.).
3) The state phase: this is dominated by the colour of the skin and mucous membranes:

- ➢ Involvement of the skin or exanthema: this is dominated by the appearance of highly itchy vesicles containing a clear liquid. These vesicles mainly affect the trunk and spare the face and limbs.
- ➢ Involvement of the mucous membranes or enanthema: here the vesicles can affect the oral mucous membranes as well as the pharynx, making it difficult to eat or suckle.

Treatment :

a) **Preventive**

- ❖ Vaccination: there is a chickenpox and shingles vaccine called VZV OKA isolated from a Japanese child called OKA

b) Curative :

- ❖ **Etiological: the** child is given acyclovir or zovirax intravenously or orally, 5mg/kg in three or two doses/10 days.

Role of the nurse :

- Isolating the child
- Treat skin, eye, nose and mouth/throat lesions with an antiseptic
- Reducing fever
- Preventing bacterial superinfection through the use of ATBs
- Reduce pruritus with an anti-histamine, e.g. phenergan
- Prescribing a sedative for insomnia

VIII.2. BACTERIAL DISEASES

Tetanus

When a child presents with trismus, muscle spasms at the slightest stimulation, hypertonia of the muscles manifested by opistotonos, or a wound, however small, the nurse's role will be to :

a) **Preventive**

- Vaccination
- Appropriate wound care;
- For neonatal tetanus: encourage births at the health centre or hospital, improve care materials and disinfection of birth areas by midwives;
- Health education for umbilical cord care (asepsis when cutting and disinfecting the cord, application of sterile dressings);
- Full vaccination of pregnant women with ANC (5 doses in total during their lifetime or childbearing years);
- Give 1500 IU of SAT to all newborns on 4^e days after delivery under suspect conditions.

b) **Curative**

- SAT
- ATB therapy, preferably penicillin;
- Care of the entry point, disinfection of the umbilicus or wound to the point of bleeding to allow air access, as C. tetani is anaerobic and dies in the presence of oxygen.
- Take care of the sick child's environment: a dark, calm and quiet room;
- Absolute rest

- Do not touch or move the child as much as possible
- Strict ban on visits
- Close monitoring of the child
- Calming the child to attenuate the seizures and not to suppress them, which would be tantamount to excessive and dangerous sedation. In this case, Diazepam, phenobarbital and largactif are used alternately as sedatives.
- Ensure fluid and food intake and, if necessary, insert an NGLS as soon as the seizures have been calmed by 1er sedative treatment;
- Don't forget to vaccinate children who have had tetanus, as they haven't Pr acquired as much immunity;
- Newborns should also be rotated every 3 hours. But never leave them on their back for long periods, as there is a danger of false swallowing. This also helps to prevent bedsores and bronchopneumonia;
- The use of a monitoring sheet here is essential to record all the actions taken.

NB**: the prognosis for** a child with tetanus depends on :

- ❖ The speed at which the treatment progresses.
- ❖ Especially the amount of nursing care.

VIII.3. PARASITIC DISEASES

Malaria: malaria is responsible for a large proportion of infant mortality in the tropics, as 1/3 of deaths before the age of one or are caused by malaria.

1) **Prevention**: prevention is one of the most important aspects of the CPS's activities.

A study of the preventive measures available and achievable locally should be carried out, leading to an **action plan** such as :

- ❖ Public health measures :
- ▪ Cleaning up the environment
- ▪ Destruction of marshes and puddles;
- ▪ Deforestation ;
- ▪ The use of an insecticide-treated mosquito net is currently recommended.
- ▪ IPT (intermittent presumptive treatment) in pregnant women consists of administering SP (three doses at ANC):
  The first dose at 16e weeks, the 2e dose at 28e weeks and the 3e dose at 32e weeks.

Teach your mother how to look after the mosquito net: do not wash it in soapy water, do not iron.

In many regions, children are exposed to malaria attacks for up to 5 years. After that, if they survive, they will have acquired immunity.

2) **Curative**

- ❖ Artesunate at a rate of : 3 mg/Kg of weight and amodiaquine 4mg/kg for 3 days.
- ❖ Quinine: 20mg/Kg in cases of severe malaria as a loading dose in 5% glucosé 20ml/kg to run for 4 hours then rest for 8 hours. The maintenance dose is 10mg/kg in G5% 10ml/kg for 4 hours.

3) Treatment of complications

Add the following specific treatment to the curative treatment below:

- Check the temperature and combat it if there is a fever;
- Check for dehydration; if necessary, start a drip;
- Monitor cerebral malaria (sedatives should be used in the event of a convulsion);
- Check for haemolytic anaemia and transfuse if necessary by measuring Hb.

CHAP. IX. ENDOCRINE DISEASES

DIABETES

The role of the nurse

a) **Insulin therapy**: nurses must be familiar with the different types of insulin, their appearance, mode of action, elimination time and all the precautions to be taken when administering this medicine.

These precautions are :

- Ensure that the patient has eaten for more than 30 minutes before administering this medicine;
- Constantly changing injection sites;
- Strict adherence to asepsis because the patient has an immune deficiency;
- Keep this medicine refrigerated;
- The use of a special insulin syringe is essential for the correct dosage of this medicine;
- The nurse must know that 1ml of insulin contains 40 I.U.

b) Monitoring the patient

It is based on glucose management, which must be carried out after every 4 hours or at least 3 times a day.

The dose will be determined by the doctor on the basis of the blood glucose level.

Other tests may be considered, such as blood glucose, acetonuria, etc.

c) Education for diabetic children and their parents.

- Inform parents and children about the diet.
- The child should be put on a suitable diet or referred to a nutritionist.
- Inform parents about the slightest warning signs that may require medical attention.

CHAP.X. MANAGEMENT OF ACUTE MALNUTRITION

X.1. INTRODUCTION

Protein-energy malnutrition occurs when a child does not get enough energy or protein from food to meet his or her nutritional needs. A child who has been frequently ill may suffer from protein-energy malnutrition, the child's appetite decreases and the food consumed by the child is poorly utilised.

When the child suffers from protein-energy malnutrition

- He may lose weight severely: a sign of sluggishness,
- There may be oedema: kwashiorkor sign
- They may not grow normally because their growth is impaired (stunted growth).

Any child whose diet does not contain the recommended quantities of essential vitamins and minerals may suffer from malnutrition.

X.2. CAUSES

There are two main groups of causes of malnutrition:

Primary and secondary causes

A. PRIMARY CAUSES OR PRIMARY AETIOLOGIES

This is essentially a quantitative and qualitative insufficiency of the various nutrients in the body.

B. SECONDARY CAUSES

Several factors are involved in the onset of malnutrition, including :

- ✓ Early weaning
- ✓ Late weaning
- ✓ Various infections of the digestive tract
- ✓ Wars and political instability
- ✓ Natural disasters
- ✓ Illiteracy, especially among mothers
- ✓ Household size

Clinically, there are two types of severe acute malnutrition: kwashiorkor and marasmus.

KWASHIORKOR	MARASME
- Pure protein deficiency - Presence of oedema - Normal or increased weight due to oedema - Size kept normal - Skin fats are preserved - Variable dermatoses (Mucous membrane and skin lesions) - He is listless and has no appetite	- It's an overall lack of energy - No oedema - Significant weight loss - Size reduction - Subcutaneous fat disappears - Little or no skin dermatitis - Appetite preserved, active.

Certain indicators enable us to distinguish between these two forms of acute-severe malnutrition, including the GOMEZ index or the WELLCOME index

a) GOMEZ index

He evaluated the normal weight for the child's age according to the following formula:

$$Poids\ pour\ l'age = \frac{Poids\ actuel\ du\ sujet\ X\ 100}{Poids\ idéal\ de\ l'enfantde\ même\ âge}$$

The result can be interpreted as follows:

Nutritional status	**Percentage**
Normal state	Between 90% and 100%.
Minor or mild malnutrition	Between 75% and 90
Moderate malnutrition	Between 60% and 75%.
Severe malnutrition	Less than 60%.

b) GOMEZ Modified or WELLCOME

He uses the same formula and interprets it as follows:

Weight for age	**Presence of oedema**	**Absence of oedema**
60 à 80%	Kwashiorkor	Undernutrition
<60%	Kwashiorkor -marasmic	Marasmus

Complications: there are two types

a) **Acute complications**
- Severe anaemia
- Severe hypoglycaemia
- Severe hypothermia
- Severe sepsis

b) **Chronic or late complications**
- Chronic malnutrition
- Delayed height and weight
- Cerebral damage, which will result in poor performance at school, clumsiness with the hands, etc.

The role of the nurse

a) **In prevention**
- Weaning should be carried out using local foodstuffs that are available and accessible at an acceptable cost to everyone at the right time.
- Correct treatment of digestive tract infections
- Recommend a sufficient and balanced diet
- Cultivating a culture of peace

b) **In the assessment of nutritional status (diagnosis) based on certain criteria :**

- **Clinical criteria**: look for nutritional oedema (bilateral, symmetrical, painless, soft, ascending) and visible, severe weight loss.
- **Anthropometric parameters** :

- Weight-for-height index: less than -3 ET in cases of severe acute malnutrition and between -2ET and -3ET in cases of moderate malnutrition.
- Brachial perimeter (BP) at MUAC: less than 115 mm in severe malnutrition and between 115 and 125 mm in moderate malnutrition

NB: lack of appetite and associated pathologies are severe complications of malnutrition.

c) In treatment

- ❖ Cases of severe acute malnutrition without complications: these cases are monitored on an outpatient basis, i.e. in the UNTA (Unité Nutritionnelle Thérapeutique Ambulatoire - Outpatient Therapeutic Nutrition Unit)
- ❖ Cases of moderate malnutrition: these are cases monitored in a UNS (therapeutic nutritional supplementation unit).

A) In an NICU (severe case with complications) :

- ✓ **Medical treatment**: treat complications by combining systematic treatment with amoxycillin, vitamin A vaccination according to EPI, albendazol and folic acid.
- ✓ **Nutritional treatment**: this is carried out in two stages: on admission, treatment is based on F75 therapeutic milk (with the exception of cases referred from UNTA for a period of observation linked to weight loss or stagnant weight for no known reason but with a retained appetite.) when the medical complications are under control and the patient's appetite has returned, the patient is switched to the ATPE to prepare him/her for treatment in the UNTA if the patient has been referred from the UNTA to the UNTI with a preserved appetite, he/she receives the ATPE directly instead of the LT.
- ✓ **Administration and preparation of LT F75:** The patient receives 100 Kcal/kg/day spread over 6 meals, i.e. every 4 hours. In some specific cases (anorexic patients, frequent vomiting, diarrhoea due to malnutrition, hypoglycaemia or recent hypothermia, etc.) the milk should be given at 8 meals. Once the complications are under control, the oedema has begun to melt and the patient's appetite has been restored, the patient should be gradually introduced to the ATPE in preparation for transfer to the UNTA. The first step is to carry out an appetite test.

B) In a case of severe acute malnutrition (UNTA)

Systematic medical treatment: oral amoxy, albenda or mebenda, vit A, ACT if malaria test **+,** vaccination.

Nutritional treatment :

Nutritional treatment in UNTA is based on ATPE (ready-to-use therapeutic food), e.g. plumpynut, BP100 5, which has the same nutritional and energy value as LT F100. ATPs must be administered to the patient as they are, without mixing them with water or other ingredients.

Instructions for using ATP at home.

RUTFs are food supplements intended only for cases of severe malnutrition where the patient (generally a child aged between 6 and 24 months) is unable to eat the RUTF or compact biscuit as it is, and the mother must prepare small quantities of porridge (neither too liquid nor too compact) with clean water for each meal.

C) Treatment in an SNU (moderate malnutrition)

Systematic medical treatment: albenda or mebenda, vit A, ACT if malaria test +, vaccination.

Nutritional treatment: the SNU ration is a supplement to the daily food ration which should not be shared between other members of the family. The dry ration should provide between 1000 and 1200 K cal/day/person. It is made up of a mixture of flour, cereals and legumes enriched with micronutrients, oils enriched with vitamin A and sugar.

CHAP. XI. URINARY AND GENITAL INFECTIONS.

A number of diseases can affect a child's urinary tract, including urinary tract infections, nephrotic syndrome, and acute and chronic renal failure.
We are particularly interested in urinary tract infections in children.

XI.1. DEFINITION

A urinary tract infection is the colonisation of a child's urine by various germs. They occur in 0.5 to 1% of premature newborns, especially boys. They affect 3% of girls under the age of 3, and 5% of school-age girls have a urinary infection at least once. This condition is often under-diagnosed in children, which increases the risk of the disease developing into chronic renal failure.
Route of contamination
There are two routes of contamination:

- The descending or haematogenous route
- The way up

a) **The descending or haematogenous route**: in this case, colonisation of the urine occurs from an infectious site in the body, where the germs leave the site, reach the bloodstream and are carried to the urinary tract. This mode of contamination is more common in newborns.
b) **The ascending route**: in this route, microbes spread from the urethra to the bladder and colonise the urine. In this route, the microbes come from faecal flora. This route of urine colonisation is more common in infants and older children.

XI .2. CONTRIBUTING FACTORS

There are many reasons for this, including the non-circumcision of infants:

- Uncircumcised children have ten times more urinary tract infections than circumcised children or girls;
- The short urethra in girls: this explains the increased incidence of urinary tract infections in girls because the short urethra is close to the rectum (faecal flora);
- The bladder does not empty completely,
- Vesico-urethral reflux (VUR): this is an anatomical defect or malformation of the uretero-vesical function that encourages urine to stagnate in the bladder, leading to the development of germs that colonise the urine;
- Some uropathogenic bacteria have the ability to adhere to the mucosa, enabling these infectious agents to travel up the urinary tract to the kidneys.

XI.3. CLINICAL SIGNS

a) In newborns

The clinical signs are non-specific, but the following signs can be observed:

- Thermal instability, especially hypothermia
- Digestive problems: vomiting and diarrhoea
- Weight loss or weight stagnation.

b) In infants aged 1 month and 2 years, we have :

- ✓ Unexplained fever (ask for a urine sedimentation test)
- ✓ Weight loss
- ✓ Digestive disorders: vomiting, diarrhoea and anorexia
- ✓ Abdominal colic (systematic stool and urine tests)
- ✓ Haematuria

c) In children over the age of two: the classic signs are as follows:

- ❖ Fever,
- ❖ Lower back pain
- ❖ Enuresis, dysuria, mictalgia, pollakiuria

The role of the nurse

- ✓ Circumventing children
- ✓ A reminder of perineal hygiene for young girls
- ✓ Ensure adequate fluid intake, and encourage parents to give the child plenty of water to drink, as this helps to fight infection by increasing diuresis.
- ✓ Encourage individual use of toilet facilities by children.
- ✓ Do urine tests and give antibiotics depending on the results?

CHAP. XII. PTME AND THE CHILD WITH HIV

XII.1 PMTCT

This is the protection of mother-to-child transmission of HIV. This is a programme set up by the National AIDS Control Programme (PNLS) to prevent HIV transmission from HIV-positive mothers to their children.

Methodology in the field, the application of PMTCT takes place at ANC sessions and follows the following stages:

- **The educational session.**

This is done at each ANC session, where pregnant women are informed about HIV/AIDS in general, HIV infection in pregnant women, PMTCT and HIV screening.

During this session, or to motivate pregnant women to take the voluntary test, a new approach has very recently been introduced: the use of image boxes.

Counselling: this is an interview/advice between a trained counsellor and the woman to prepare her to accept the test and the result.

This interview takes place before and after the test, and is known as pre- and post-test counselling.

Once the customer has agreed to take the test, the advisor takes a blood sample for examination (2ml of venous blood).

- **The test:** The examination is carried out in the lab without knowing the woman's name, as samples are sent to the lab with numbers only.
- **Post-test counselling** or withdrawal of results. There is a further interview before the results are given.

Monitoring and preventing transmission

Pregnant women who are seropositive are monitored by the consultant, and their delivery and breastfeeding must include the following special features:

- The woman should receive **Niverapine** during labour in a single dose of one Co ;
- Newborn babies should also receive niverapine drops (2 drops/Kg) within 72 hours of birth;
- Breastfeeding will be exclusive and weaning will take place after 6 months;
- If there are lesions on the nipple or in the child's mouth, we will stop feeding even before the child is 6 months old, as lesions are a risk of contamination.
- The child of an HIV-positive mother will be tested for HIV at 18 months to see if he or she has been infected. Before 18 months, it is difficult to confirm HIV in the child of an HIV-positive mother, as the child has anti-HIV antibodies from the mother. This means that the test is always positive before 18 months, once these antibodies have been eliminated and the child has not been infected, the test will be negative after 18 months.

XII.2. CHILDREN AND HIV

AIDS is Acquired Immune Deficiency Syndrome.

Most cases are seen in adults, but paediatric AIDS is becoming increasingly common.

a) **Etiology**: the human immunodeficiency virus is the cause of this disease, and transmission is :

- ✓ Maternal fetus: 5 to 10 women in different regions of the Congo are infected. 1/3 of children born to infected mothers are also infected;
- ✓ **Transfusion**
- ✓ Injections or other procedures such as scarification
- ✓ Sexual: possible in adolescents, although common in adults.

b) **Clinic**

- ✓ The incubation period varies from a few weeks to several years (on average 1 to 2 years).
- ✓ Reduced growth, chronic diarrhoea, chronic fever, opportunistic infections (oral candidiasis resistant to treatment)

c) Diagnosis

Not to be confused with TBC and other forms of malnutrition. Clinical GD is confirmed by finding 2 major signs and 2 minor signs.
In paediatrics, the major signs include:

- Slower growth ;
- Diarrhoea lasting more than a month.
- Chronic fever

Minor signs

- Generalised lymphadenopathy
- Candidiasis
- Repeated common infections
- Cough for more than a month

d) Treatment

- Preventing modes of transmission
- Mothers can transmit HIV through breast milk, so if artificial milk is available, it can be used instead of breast milk;
- Treatment of women during labour can reduce foetomaternal transmission (niverapine). However, this drug is rarely available.
- Even if there is no possible treatment, it is useful to improve nutrition and treat other associated infections.

BIBLIOGRAPHY

1. Athreya B.H, Silverman B.K., Spitzer A.R.Semeiotica pediatrica
Masson S.p.A, Milan, 1988

2. Barness L. A Manual of clinical diagnosis in paediatrics
5ème Edition, Maloine, Paris, 1982

3. Cornu G., Malvaux P. Paediatric semiology
Syllabus UCL-Faculty of Medicine
Volunteer printing centre, Brussels, 1985-1986

4. Behrmann R.E., Kliegman R.M., Jenson H.B.Nelson Textbook of Pediatrics
16th Edition, Saunders, Philadelphia, 2000

5. Forfar J.O, Arneil G.C. Textbook of Paediatrics
Vol.2, 3rd Edition, Langman Group Limited
Edinburgh, 1984

6. The state of the world's children 2003
Official summary, UNICEF

7. National survey on the situation of children and women
DRC/ UNICEF/ USAID analysis report
Kinshasa, July 2002

8. Espérance K, course notes in Paediatric Nursing, ISTM-GOMA 2021

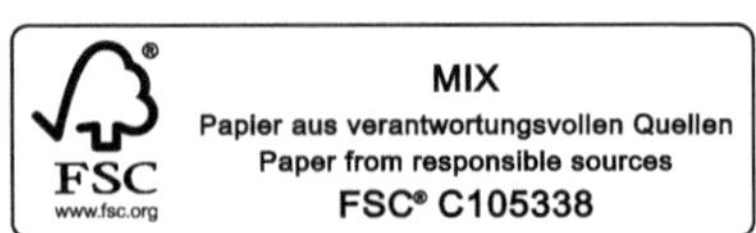

Printed by Books on Demand GmbH, Norderstedt / Germany